SCIENCE AT WORK
FACE FACTS

A R KENNEY

NELSON

Who needs camouflage?

Your changing skin

When you were a toddler the skin over your whole body looked lovely. It has changed since then: the palms of your hands and the soles of your feet have hardened, thickened and coarsened; on your arms and legs it is a shade less pliant and your face, although attractive, may well now be blemished. Gradually the skin loses its child-like softness as a result of the ravages of sun, rain, strong and icy winds or even the accidental scratches and abrasions of everyday life. It is only the covered skin that retains its loveliness until old age.

Using cosmetics

Elsewhere the skin changes with time. It will coarsen where it is most exposed, it may become greasy or dry and flakey, it will certainly gain wrinkles and stretch a little — the young child's natural skin beauty will very slowly fade away. How quickly this happens will depend on the individual. But for most women, and more recently for men, cosmetics are used to protect the skin from the sun and wind and to help the skin retain its youthful appearance.

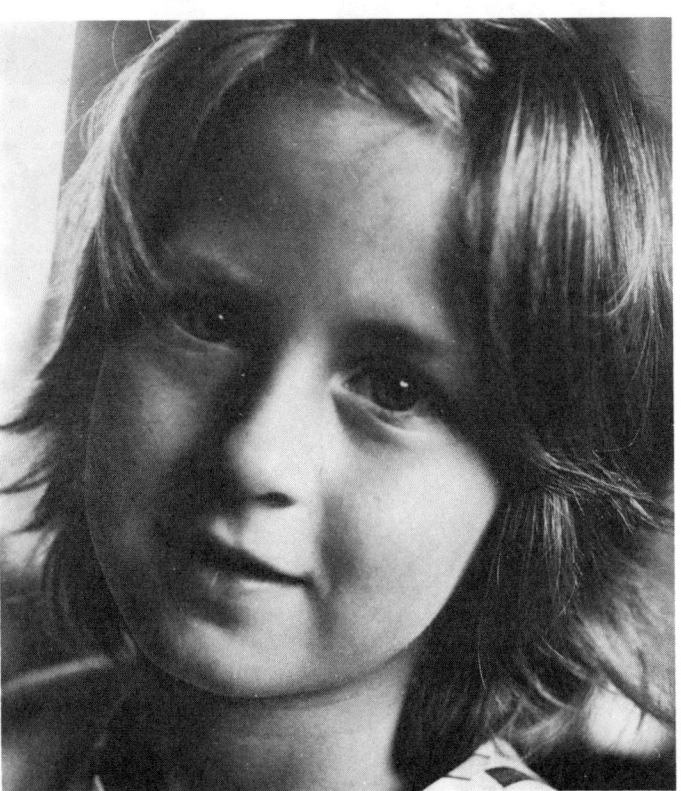

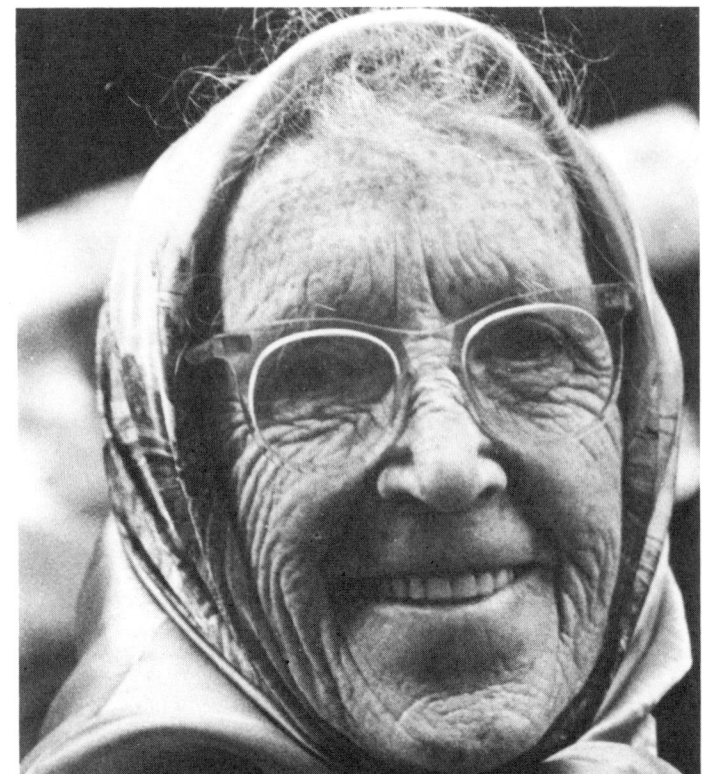

Cosmetics long ago

This use of cosmetics is by no means a new phenomenon. It isn't even associated with 'civilization' or a wealthy society. There is evidence that men and presumably women decorated their bodies with paints away back in prehistoric times. The ancient **Egyptians** used 'cosmetics', and in **Elizabethan times** the women washed their faces in red wine to give them ruddy complexions. Some African tribes do the same thing: a war dance would lose much character if performed by undecorated naked bodies and, likewise, festival dances depend to a large extent on the accessories of paints, bangles, costumes and feathers.

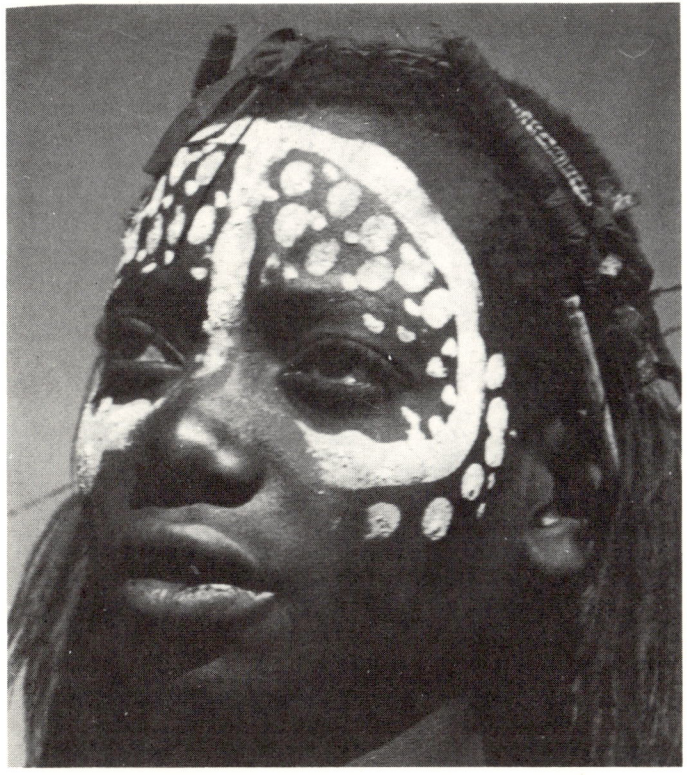

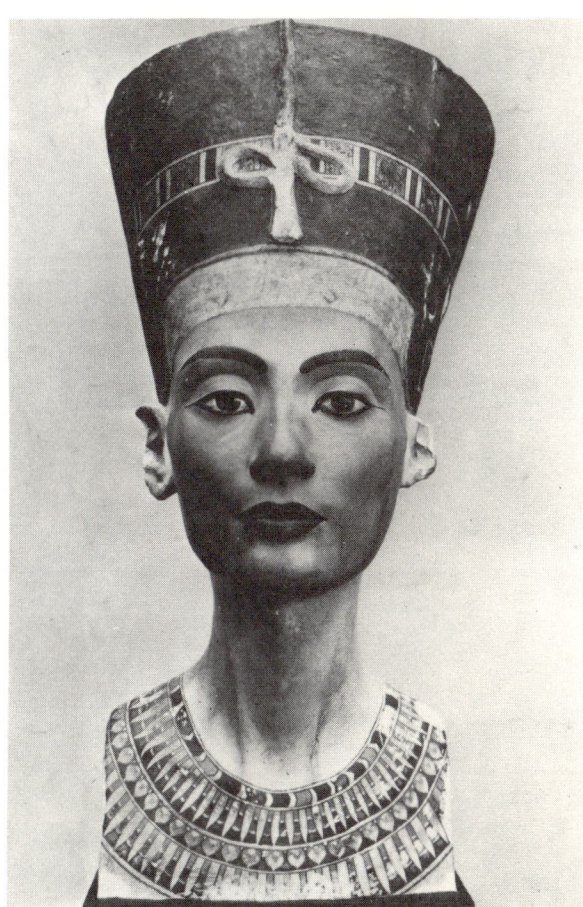

Camouflage

In a way, the use of cosmetics, and, indeed, fashionable clothes, are an attempt to deceive the viewer into believing that the performer has greater powers, is more beautiful, more strong, more awe-inspiring, than he or she really is. By adding a high feather head dress over their heads, warriors appear to be taller, and therefore stronger, than they really are. Cosmetics could be described as a type of **camouflage**.

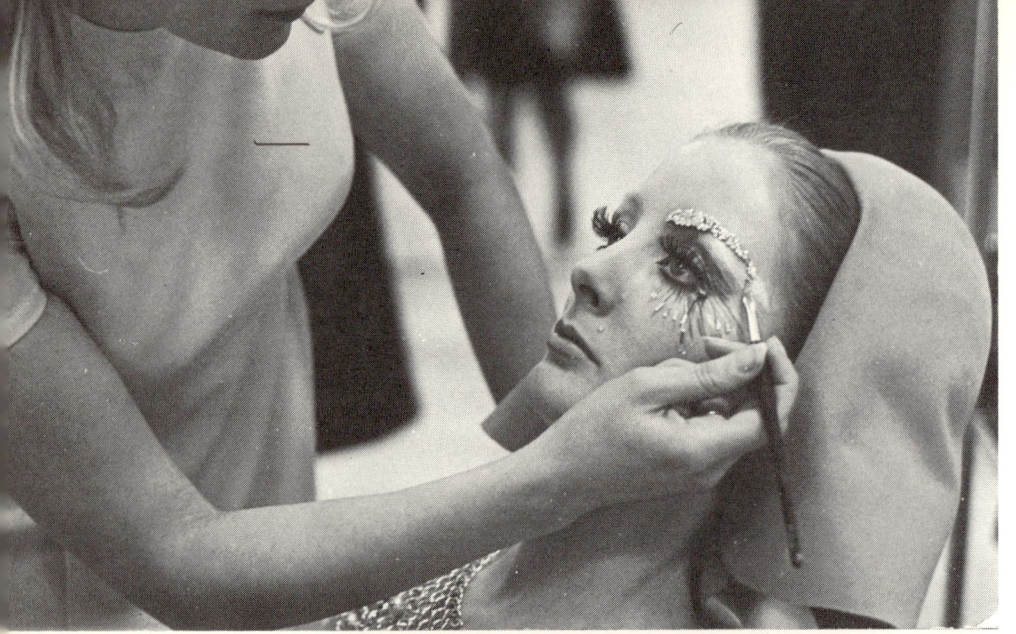

There are occasions when cosmetics are used to highlight good features but just as often the cosmetic can help to play down or even cover up the poor skin.

Camouflage is important in the animal kingdom too:

Using cosmetics for protection

In the animal world the eye is of such importance that it is the natural target for attack. As a protection, some animals camouflage the eye by colouring and recessing it and then, behind the head, have a mark which resembles an eye. If the latter is attacked no harm comes to the animal.

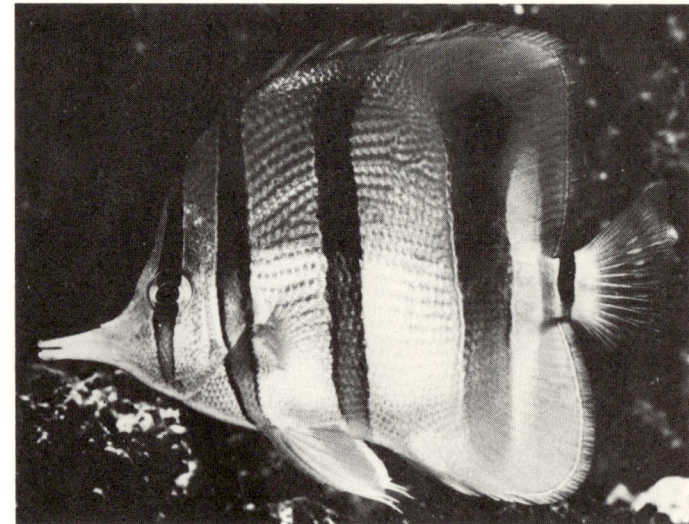

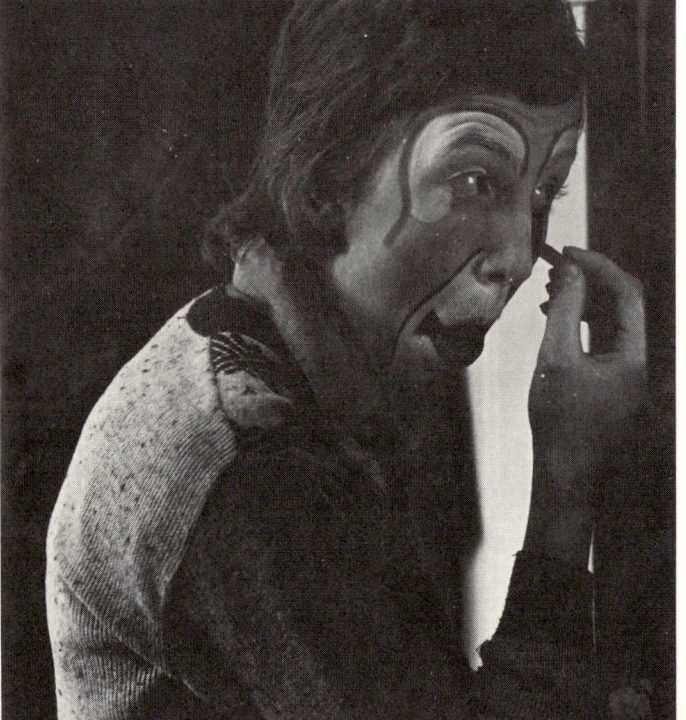

Where the animal is strong, the eye is sometimes accentuated rather than camouflaged and so in tribal decoration huge rings are painted round the eyes in an attempt to dominate the foe. Apart from the effect on the foe there is also some self deception: if one appears to be taller and if one's face looks more aggressive than it really is, then one can gain a feeling of confidence when facing the foe.

Courtship behaviour

Competition in everyday life is of great importance, but basically there is a more important biological force. Biologists call it **'The perpetuation of the species'**, in other words the reproduction of one generation to form the next. Each animal lives its life and to the individual its life may seem important. What is far more important, biologically, is the whole species, all the millions of animals of the same kind one generation following another.

You've probably heard of the 'Save the Wild Life Fund', which is an organization set up to try to preserve wild animals in danger of extinction. In the case of some animals, for example, the white rhinoceros, the total numbers are minimal and their chances of reproducing are so reduced that in a decade some could have gone for ever. It is of prime importance, therefore, that each generation of animals, whether moths, slugs, lions or man produces another generation. Nature's way of achieving this is by arranging for a male and female to come together and copulate. But when you think about it, why should a moth which has lived all its life alone suddenly decide to join another moth so that sperm can be transferred from one to the other? Birds are more gregarious, that is they tend to live in groups for at least part of their lives, but even so why does one peacock mate with a particular peahen?

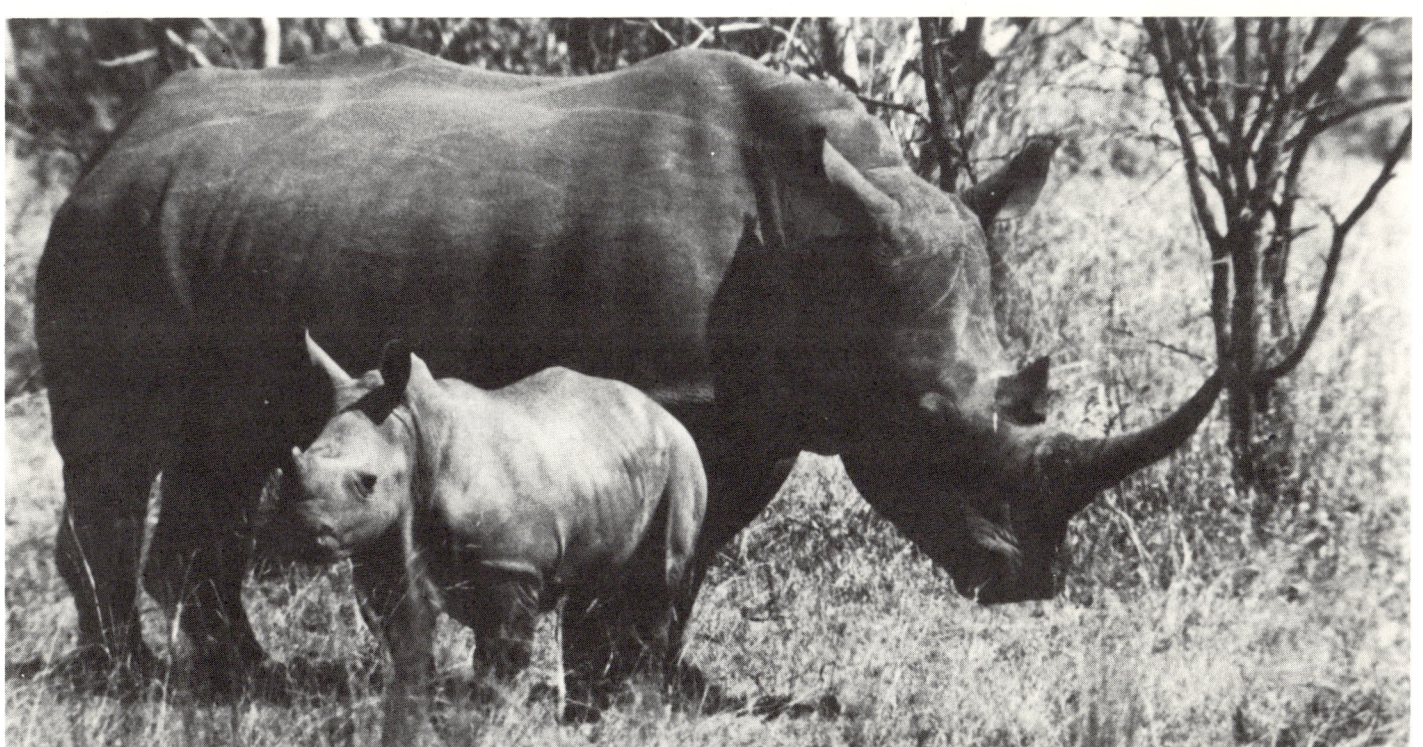

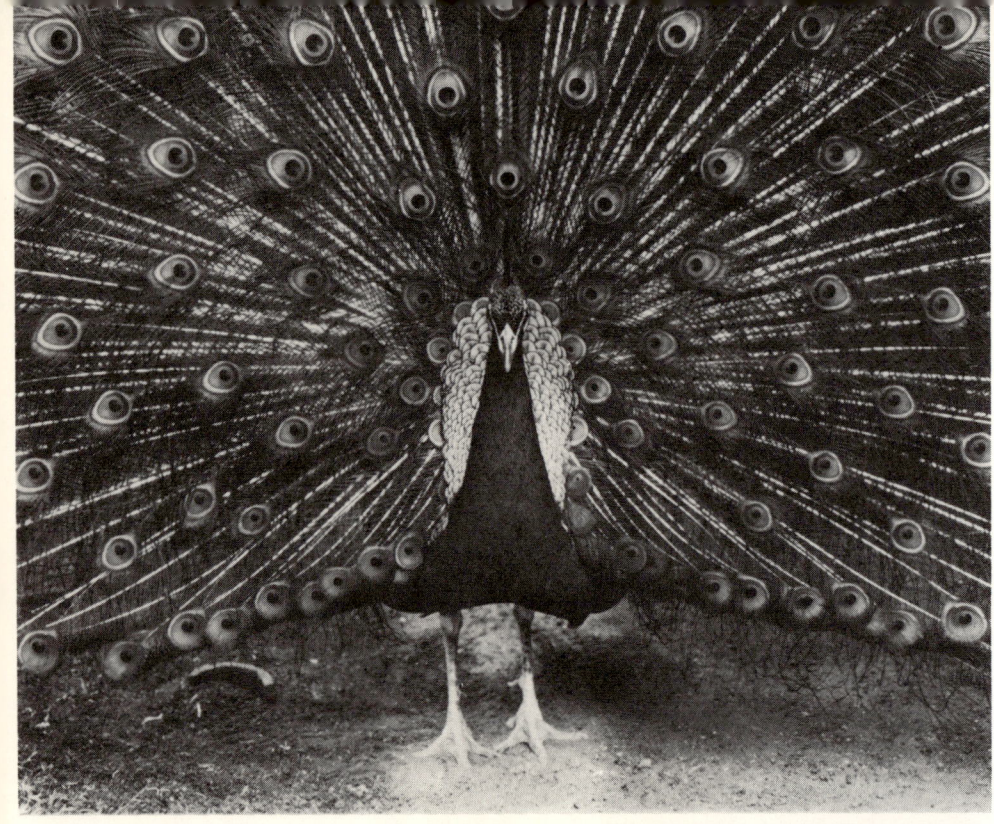

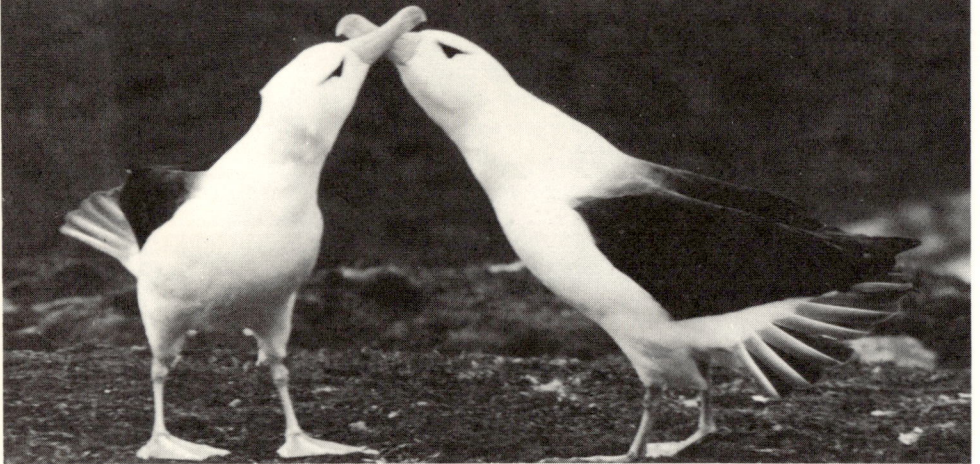

Courtship in animals

There has been much research on mating behaviour in animals and certain things have emerged as factors which lead up to mating in the animal world.

1. **Shape** plays a very important part: although monkeys and man are of similar shape, both monkeys and man know which is which.
2. **Colour and decoration:** different species have particular colour patterns. A familiar example of this is the tail of a peacock which is fanned out during premating courtship; and just think of butterflies.
3. **Movement:** in some cases partners in mating react to special patterns of movement. An example is the **fiddler crab**. There are several species of this crab to be found on the seashore and each species only mates with its own kind. The male and female recognize each other by the pattern and timing of waving movements of the front claws. This is so precise as to be absolutely accurate for identification. Next time you are in a place such as a city centre and are surrounded by **pigeons** watch them closely. Probably you will see one pigeon following another with his head and tail close to the ground. Yes, it is a 'he' and it is a male pigeon courting a female. The head and tail dipping is an essential part of his display if he is to gain the female's attention.
4. **Scent:** chemical scents are tremendously important in inter-animal relationships. Not a great deal had been discovered about scents until recently because of the difficulty of the research involved. The scents are in infinitely small quantities and it needs great expertise and complicated equipment to collect and analyse them. However, such facilities are available today and it has been proved that a female **moth** at night can attract a male from about three kilometres away (two miles) by means of scent. Scientists call these particular scents **pheromones** but scent is a perfectly good word. More recently, it has been shown that such attracting scents are to be found elsewhere in the animal world and almost certainly in man. Definitely the human male and female react to specific odours such as boar-scent.

What about humans?

Why include all this in a book about cosmetics? The answer is fairly obvious. After adolescence there is a natural affinity or getting together between boys and girls which continues right on into old age. Certain things such as shape, colouring, actions and scents tend to turn people on. A pretty red head may be one man's dream of a perfect mate but doesn't cause another man the slightest second glance. His idea of perfection could well be an oval face with rather angular cheek and jaw bones.

Women have views about the men they wish to go out with: 'tall, dark and handsome' isn't every woman's perfect man. Given, therefore, that there are basic features which cause two people to find one another attractive, then the cosmetic industry tries to accentuate and enhance the best in people and to hide away their blemishes.

Uncared for skin, broken nails and dull, unwashed hair does not help either a man or woman to seem attractive.

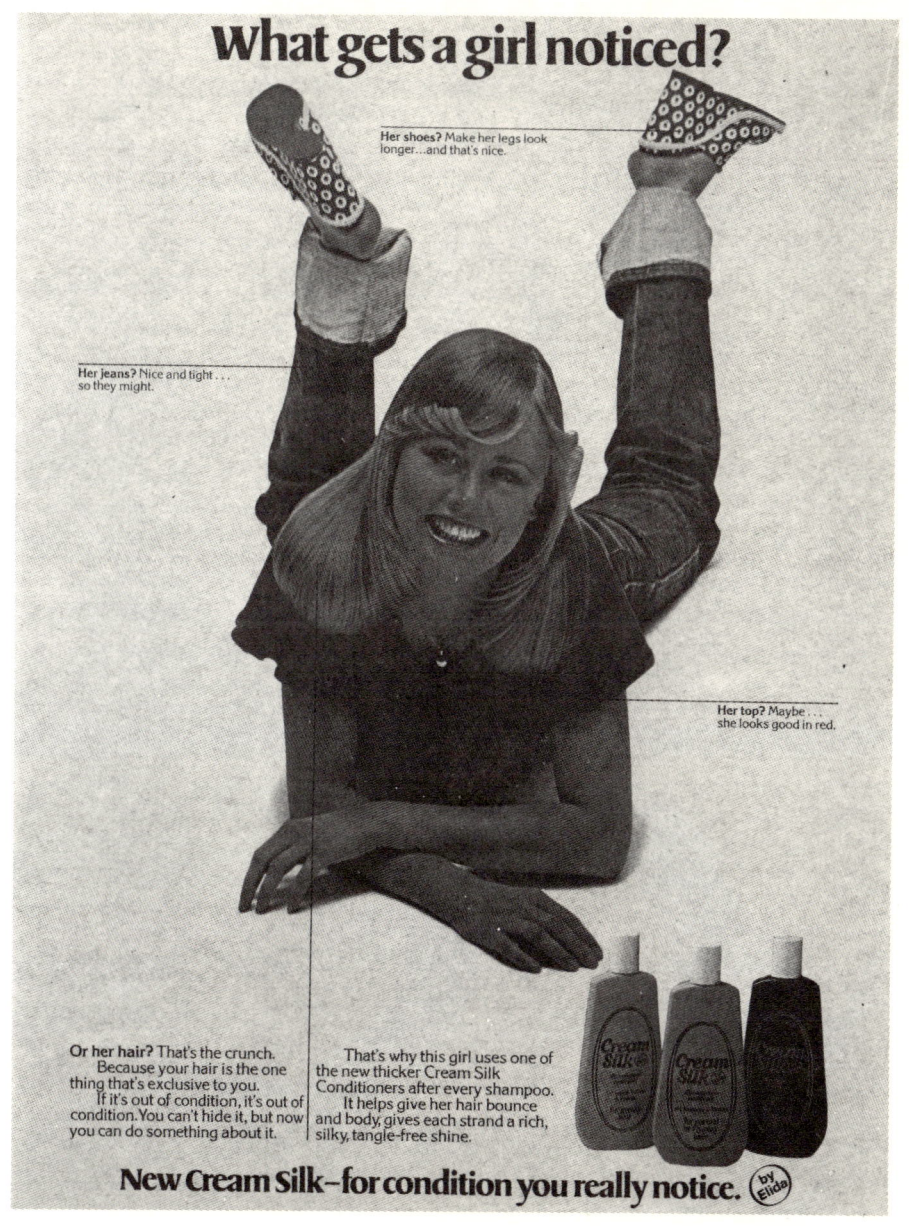

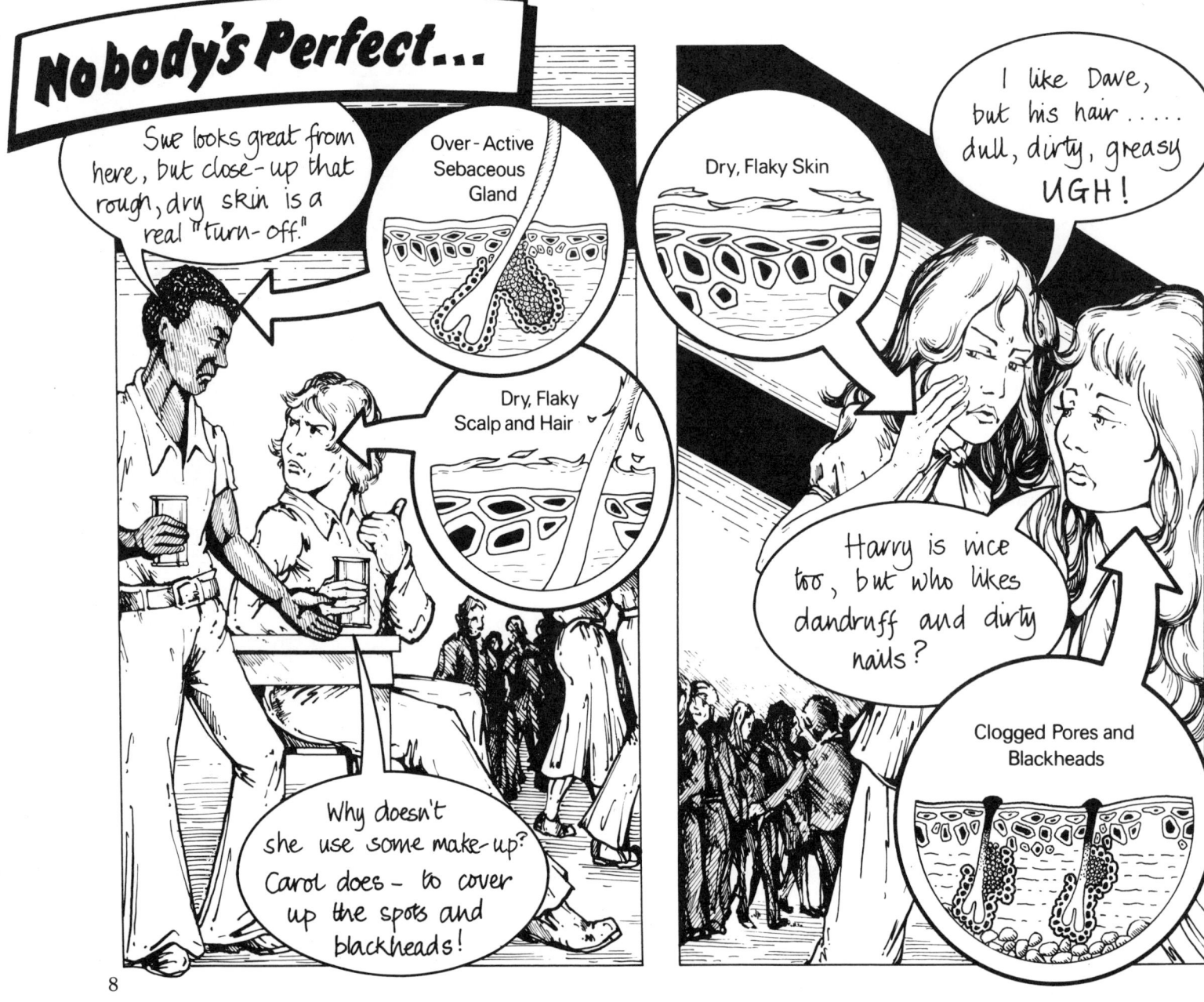

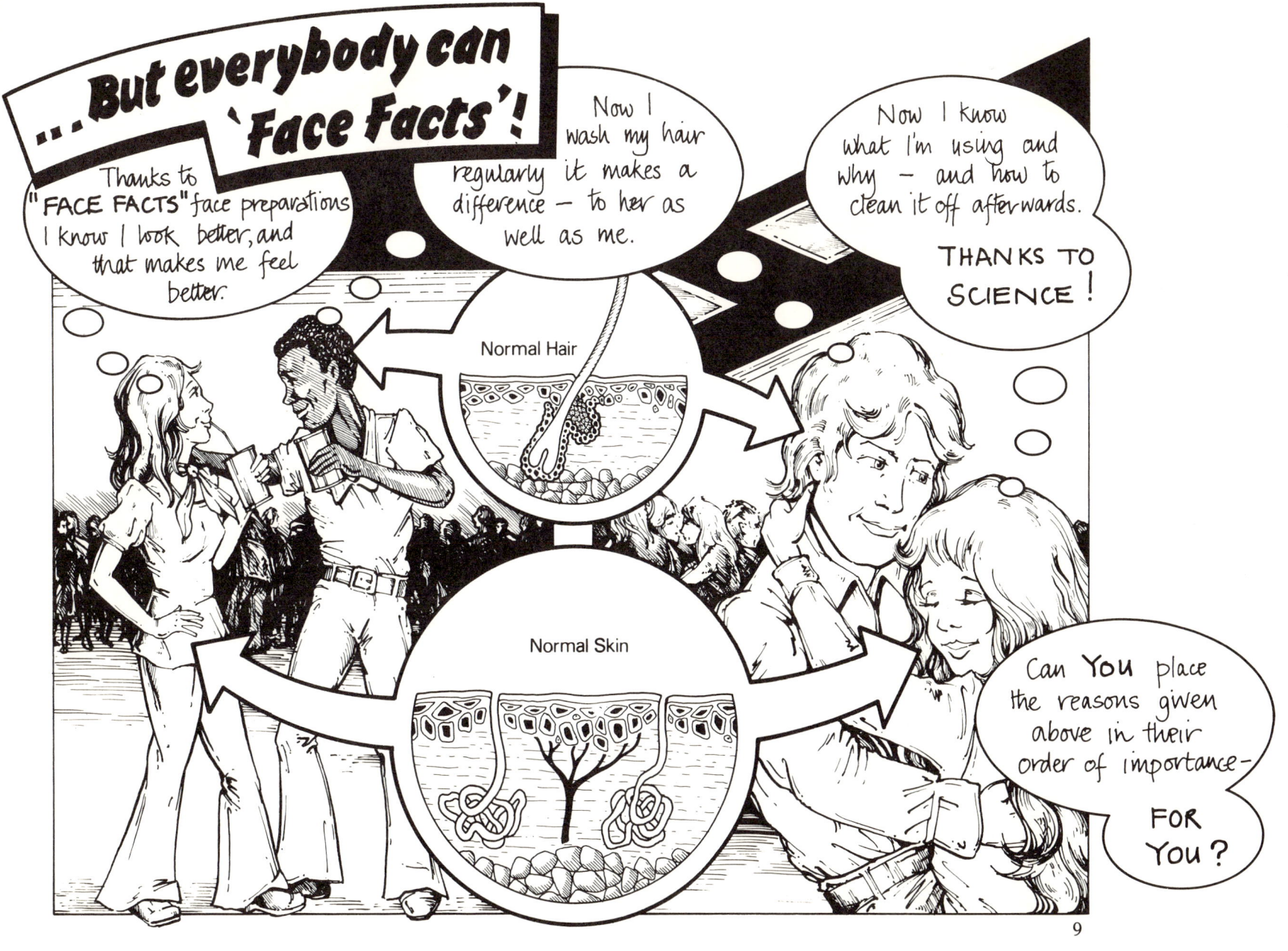

Your skin and hair

The first cosmetics

Until quite recently there was hardly any cosmetic industry at all. Nearly all creams and lotions were made at home on the kitchen stove. By the sound of the recipes many such concoctions were far from pleasant to use, nor indeed were these safe.

Safety measures

In the 1960s medical research revealed a substantial danger to health from lead metal and its compounds. In earlier centuries and without this knowledge face powders were based upon white lead with disastrous results — the beauty queens lost all their beauty and were quite haggard by the age of thirty.

Other lotions contained oils and fats which went bad: hair styles and hair dressings were so complex that, once set in place with lard and the like, they were left without further attention for weeks. Naturally the lard went rancid and the mass of hair provided nesting grounds for many insects besides lice. It wasn't unknown for mice to burrow into the hair-do during the night and make their home! No wonder both men and women had to drench themselves with scents; but as washing wasn't very popular these became stale too!

Cosmetics for all

During previous centuries the majority of the population had neither the money for cosmetics nor the leisure time to make and use them; the use of cosmetics was therefore mostly confined to high society. The past fifty years, however, have seen dramatic changes in living conditions and life styles: more people have more money and more leisure and we now realise that cosmetics can have a psychological function as well as a decorative one. In other words because cosmetics can make you look better they can also make you feel better.

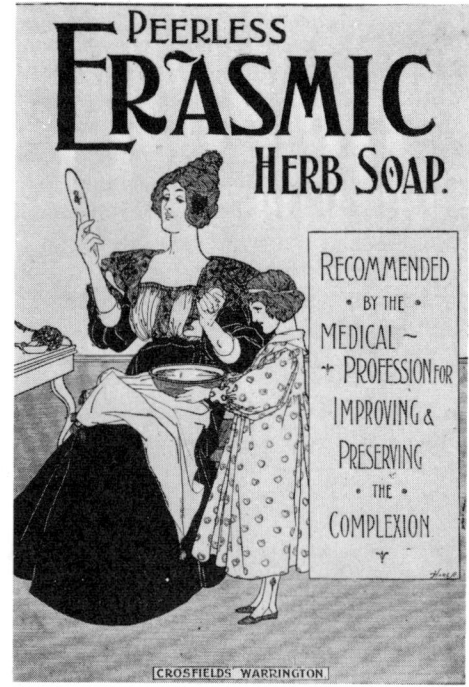

As improvements occurred in the manufacture of cosmetics, so more people started to use them in larger quantities. Home manufacture still occurred but demand was sufficient to make factory production economic.

Science and cosmetics

Apart from economics factory production had a second good result. Qualified scientists were hired to advise manufacturers. They were made responsible for knowing about skin, nail and hair structure and for knowing about which chemicals would be safe and beneficial to the user. As we shall see later the head chemist in a factory is in a key position and has great authority as to what may or may not be done, regardless of the demands of commerce.

Starting with skin

But let's look at the skin, nails and hair so that we know what we are dealing with.

1 Apart from the obvious openings into the body **our skin completely encloses us:** it seals in all our blood and fluids, and supports all the solid structures against our bony skeletons. It also keeps all other things out; dirt and germs usually stay on its surface and water normally rolls off. It takes all the knocks of everyday life in its stride, mostly without us realising it, and very important indeed, it protects us from the ultra-violet light of the sun.

All these are rather negative functions of the skin but in addition it does positive things as well.

2 **Perspiration** is something that goes on most of the time: sometimes it's very obvious on a hot day but at other times we are barely aware of it except for such places as under the arms. The sweat glands which produce perspiration are found fairly deep in the skin and can be switched on and off according to the needs of the body. They open on to the skin surface via a duct and sometimes bacteria crawl down this duct where they multiply and, in a small percentage of people, cause body odour. The control of this condition is difficult because the bacteria are hidden and fairly immune to attack.

3 We also gain a lot of **information via the skin** because many **sense organs** are embedded in it. We know when the air is warm or cold and if we touch anything hot we yell. We know when things are soft or hard, smooth or rough, blunt or sharp. We suffer pain if we are hit hard or burn ourselves; this may not seem an advantage but think of the damage which would occur if a burning cigarette between the fingers was not noticed.

4 Also important among the skin's function is its manufacture of a vital hormone **calciferol** which, until recently, was known as Vitamin D. Without it our bones wouldn't develop properly.

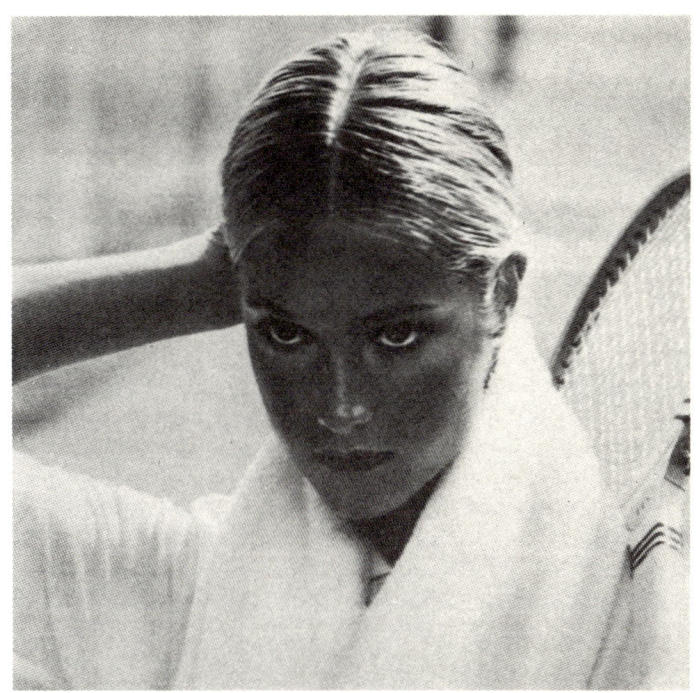

Bio Clear offers you clear, clear, beautiful skin.

The Science Of It: BIO-CLEAR medicated products have been created especially for young people with oily, troubled skin. Nowhere else will you find a complete system of integrated treatments so effective for boys and girls with problem skin.

Many of these medicated products, like the remarkable Medicated Cream, contain organic sulphide. This very effective ingredient absorbs excess oil and helps dry up blackheads, blemishes…and everything you never wanted on your skin!

The Beauty Of It: Medicated BIO-CLEAR means more than better skin. It takes away pain and embarrassment, and the fear of face-to-face confrontation. Start using BIO-CLEAR, and things will start looking up.

Free! Bring this coupon to a Helena Rubinstein consultant store. It entitles you to:
- A Beauty Consultation
- A Beauty Treatment Handbook
- A Bio Clear Product with any Bio Clear purchase

While stocks last

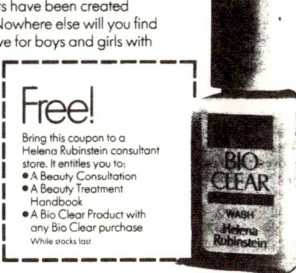

Helena Rubinstein/The Science of Beauty

Also available in Eire.

Structure of the skin

If you did not know it before, you would probably agree that the skin is important, and in the figure below you can see a cross section through the skin showing that it's made up of two main regions, the **dermis** and **epidermis**. The dermis is living and contains all the blood vessels, sweat glands and nerve endings.

The **epidermis** is dead and is made up of dead cells that started life as part of the dermis. Gradually these worked their way to the surface and became the scaly, tough outer part of the skin. Every time you touch anything or brush up against something you leave behind hundreds of dead cells. The dermis continues to make cells all through your life and because of this the epidermis is also renewed to replace the lost cells.

Greasy skin and spots

Apart from colour, we vary from person to person in the type of skin we possess and to a large extent this depends on the oily or **sebaceous glands**. These glands lubricate the skin with **sebum** and keep it supple and pliable. If the glands dry up then the skin tends to crack and become flaky and if they produce too much sebum then the skin has a shiny appearance all day — hence the shiny nose! Very often when the sebaceous glands are over active, particularly during teenage adolescence, the ducts or tubes from the glands get blocked, the oil hardens and then blackheads develop. If the right sort of bacteria get behind the blackheads then the pore and duct become septic and acne ensues.

Your skin type

So what sort of skin have you? Read through the following list because, from the cosmetic point of view, manufacturers make their products to cater for differing skin complexions and you need to buy the right ones.

1 Dry
Does your skin always appear dry and maybe slightly flaky under normal conditions?

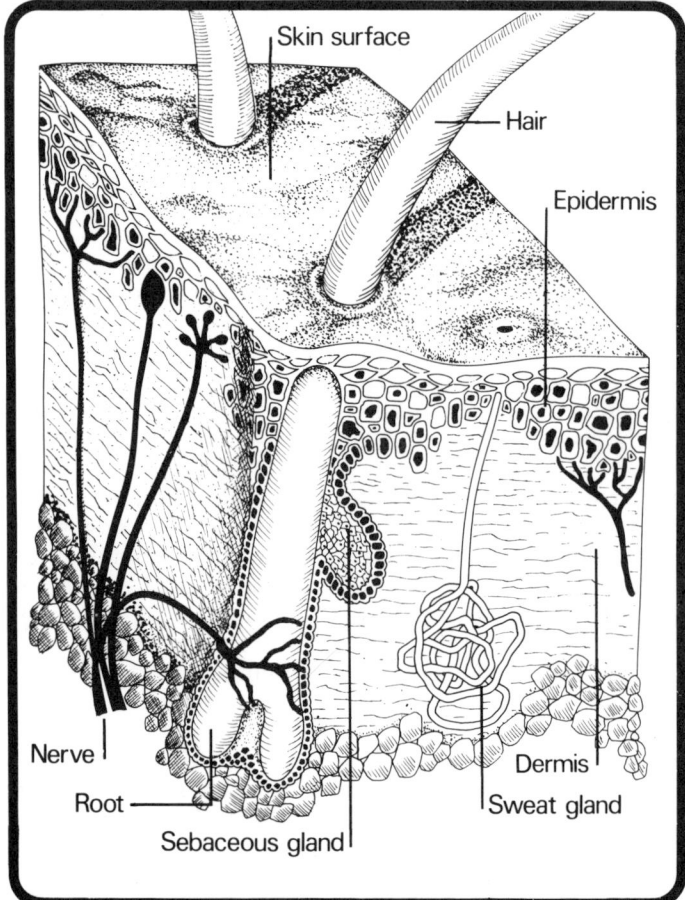

2 Oily
Does your skin often have a shiny appearance and particularly on the face? Does your hair become greasy soon after washing it?

3 In between
Is your skin neither dry nor oily? If so, you are the lucky one and your sebaceous glands are doing exactly what they should.

There are other skin types but these three are the most usual and important, and you will find products like shampoos designed for the greasy hair, dry hair and normal hair.

Now for hair

All over your body, apart from the palms of the hand and soles of the feet there are millions of hairs which grow through the **dermis** and **epidermis** from a root below.

If ever you've pulled a hair out you will have found a **root** at its base. The sebaceous gland duct opens into the tunnel surrounding the hair so that the sebum flows directly onto it. This is why people who tend to have greasy skin also have a tendency towards greasy hair.

Does your hair curl?
The hair itself is cylindrical and in cross section may be circular or oval. Circular hairs cause straight hair and oval hairs are naturally curly. Inside the cylinder is a colouring pigment which may be lost in later life, and then the hair turns grey. The surface of a hair is rather like a tiled roof. Under a microscope one can see the surface made up from hundreds of overlapping scales and if these are roughed up then one's hair looks dull.

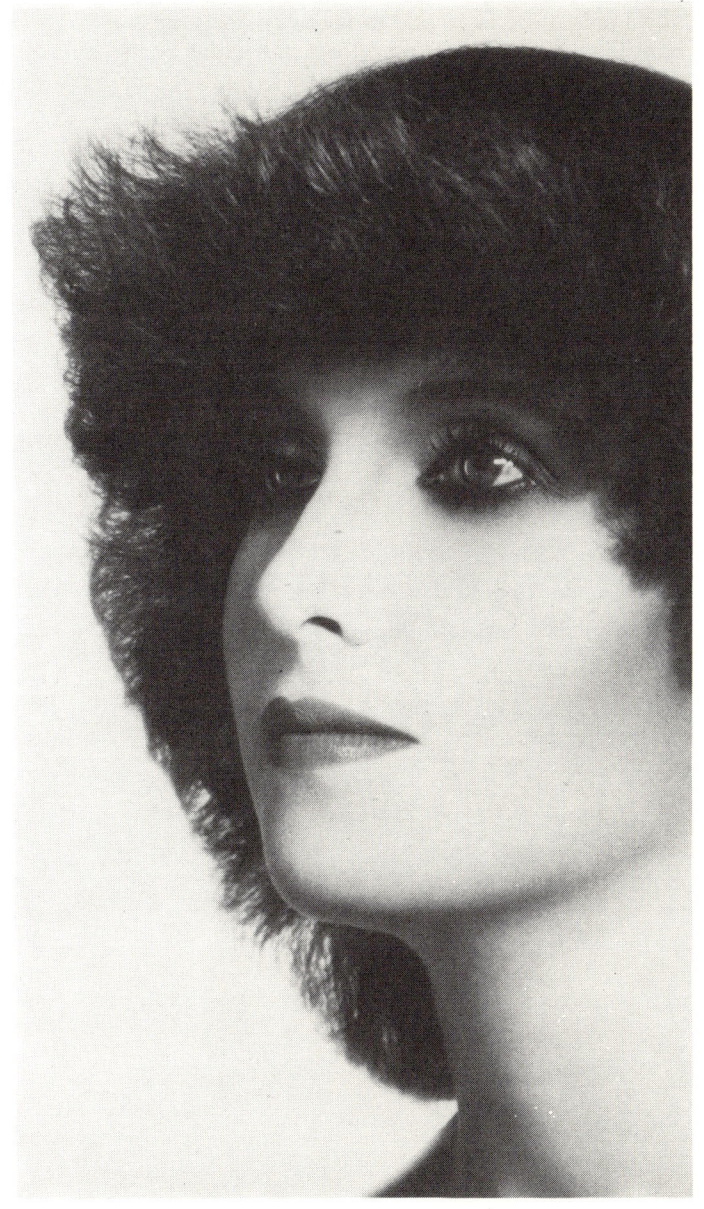

Different types of cosmetics

Nowadays there is a wide range of cosmetic products each manufactured and designed for a particular purpose. Let's look at some of them.

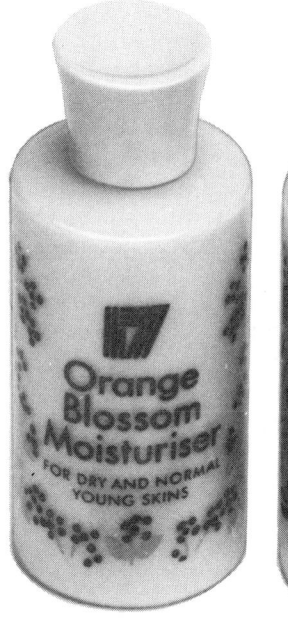
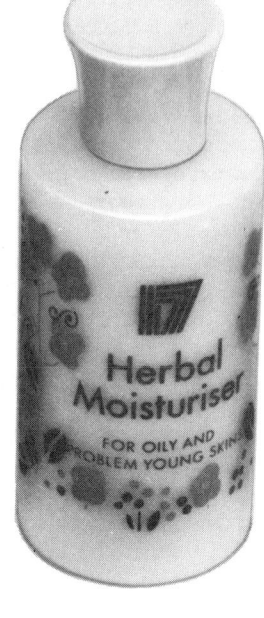
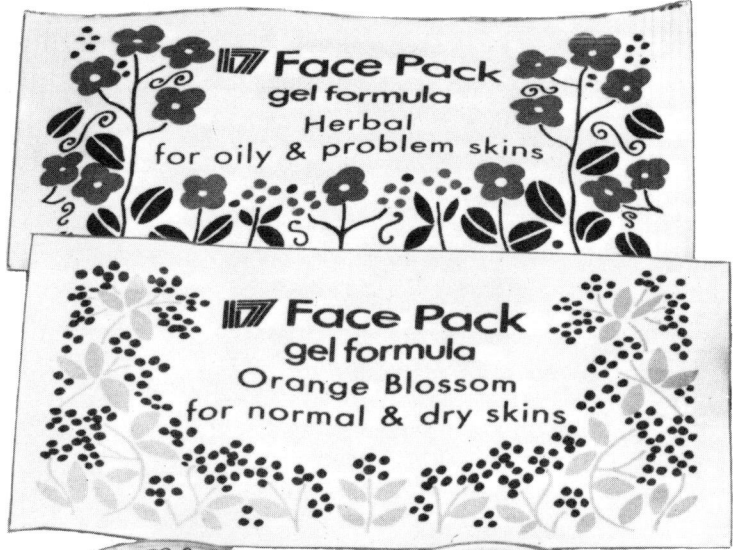

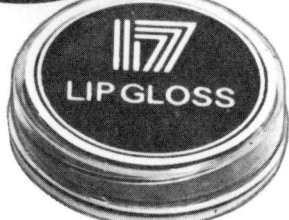

Cosmetics are divided into different categories as follows:

Skin cleaners

Soap and **water** head the list here and largely there is no cheap alternative for removing everyday grease and dirt from the skin. However, there are circumstances when it may be desirable to use a **cleansing cream** or milk as, for example, when make-up has to be removed from the eyes or perhaps where there is sensitivity or allergy to soap.

Cleansing creams and milks are essentially similar, one being a thicker edition of the other. They act by dissolving the fats of cosmetics or the natural fats of the skin in the oil within the cream or milk. Once dissolved, a paper tissue will cleanly remove everything from the skin. Cleansing creams are by no means essential for the skin and much soap is sold, some of which is very expensive and specially designed not to harm the skin.

Skin moisturizers

Rough dry skin is not a good basis for cosmetics; if one's hands are rough this can also be annoying as they catch on fine garments and cloth. The reason for the roughness is that the outer layers of the skin are too dry and lose too much water to the atmosphere. The skin is losing water all the time and, therefore, if some of the natural water is artificially retained then the skin will become moist and soft. This is the basis of most moisturisers.

'Glycerine and rose water' used to be considered a good moisturiser but now we know that it tends to extract water from the skin rather than retain it and better products are made which form a barrier between the air and skin. Water passing through the skin meets the barrier and doesn't evaporate from its surface straight away. The usual barrier is an oil and for convenience of use this is made into an emulsion with water. After application to the skin, rubbing or massaging causes it to disappear but, in fact, a very thin film of oil remains to keep the water in.

ALWAYS YOUNG!

ALWAYS FAIR!

KEEPS THE SKIN COOL AND REFRESHED IN THE HOTTEST WEATHER.

—:o:—

Beware of Injurious Imitations. '**BEETHAM'S**' is the Original and Only Genuine.

Beetham's Glycerine and Cucumber

For the Skin

THE QUEEN OF TOILET PREPARATIONS
FOR ALL SEASONS.

IS UNEQUALLED DURING THE

SUMMER MONTHS

For Preserving the Complexion from the Effects of the

HOT SUN; WINDS, HARD WATER, &c.

IT ENTIRELY REMOVES AND PREVENTS ALL

SUNBURN, REDNESS, IRRITATION, TAN,

AND RENDERS THE SKIN DELICATELY

SOFT, SMOOTH, AND WHITE.

The wonderfully Cooling Properties of the CUCUMBER JUICE render it delightfully Refreshing and Soothing if applied after being out in the Hot Sun.

TENNIS-PLAYING, WALKING, YACHTING, &c.

It allays all Irritation from the Bites and Stings of Insects. It is the most perfect Emollient Milk for the Skin ever produced, and being perfectly harmless, is INVALUABLE for the TOILET and the NURSERY. Bottles, **1s.** and **2s. 6d.**, of all Chemists. Free for 3d. extra by the Makers,

M. BEETHAM & SON, Chemists, Cheltenham.

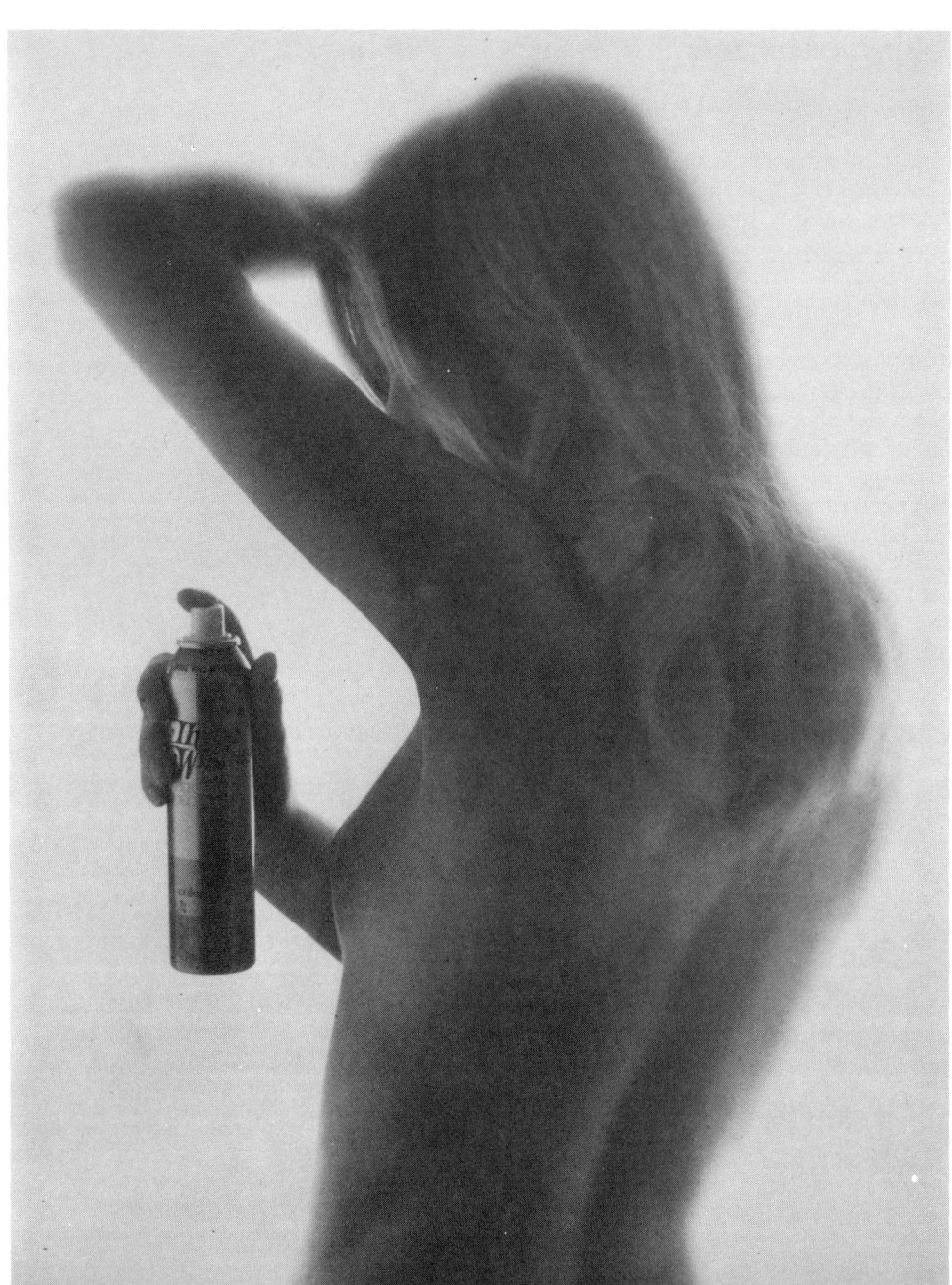

Anti-perspirants and deodorisers

Our attractiveness to others certainly drops if we smell unpleasant — hence the liberal use of scents in former centuries. Nowadays we know more about the causes of odour and can do something about it. A regular bath or shower can solve a lot of problems, but, in addition, anti-perspirants and deodorisers have a part to play.

Why do we sweat?

Perspiration is absolutely essential to a healthy body. Without it we would overheat and die. Perspiration itself is totally unscented but in time bacteria act on it and the by-product is a nasty smell. Most perspiration evaporates immediately and so there is no problem, but in certain places, for example under the arm, it remains wet and the bacteria get to work. If we use antiperspirants in these places we can reduce the secretion by 15 per cent and thus reduce the problem. Most antiperspirants are based on an aluminium salt and are applied by cloth, roll-on balls, or sprays.

How do deodorants work?

The deodoriser contains a chemical which is lethal to bacteria and by reducing their numbers smell is reduced too. Usually deodorisers are scented which adds a pleasant fragrance to the skin. Talcum powder, based on chalk or kaolin, absorbs water and quite frequently has deodorants and antiperspirants added.

Shampoos

Cleanliness of the hair is just as essential for looking great as cleanliness of the body. Soap and water removes grease and dirt but tends to leave a film over the surface of the hair so that it looks dull.

A good shampoo is rather like washing-up liquid. It's a very soft detergent which acts quickly and can be washed off easily. (Indeed some washing-up liquids make good and cheap shampoos.) However, proper shampoos include other things such as chemicals to combat dandruff (flakes of skin in the hair) or special conditioners for the hair especially suitable for those with dry or oily skins.

After-shampoo treatments

There are many hair treatments but most have the basic intention to make the hair remain in an attractive and acceptable position. **Waving** or **straightening** is achieved by heat or chemicals which unlink the natural chemical bonds within the hair and re-link these anew in the desired way. Some are permanent and others temporary.

Various resin-based **sprays** are used which dry out and hold the hair in a given style. Men now use these kind of sprays although brilliantines and creams still have a good market for the same purpose.

Some hair requires rather different care. Do you remember how the outside of a hair is covered with tiny scales? These can be distorted from their usual pattern and need **conditioners** to return them into place.

So far we have seen what might be called the basic materials which put the skin and hair into a favourable condition for make-up or the improvement of one's natural features. There are several products which enhance our good looks. They are summarised in the following table which tells you what the various products contain and what they do.

Type of Make-up	Composition	Use
1 Foundation Cream	An emulsion of oil in water.	Provides a film over the skin surface on which other cosmetics will spread evenly.
2 Powder	Talc, kaolin, chalk together with various metallic salts, colouring and scent.	Absorption of moisture from the skin, camouflaging of skin blemishes and generally improving appearance.
3 Blushers	A distinctive colouring matter, e.g. rouge, which is spread by a powder or liquid.	A blush can appear to alter the shape of the face by highlighting special features such as the cheek bones. Because blushes carry stronger colours than powders they can be used in contrast.
4 Lipstick	Mainly fat but with additives to help spreading and adhesion. It has to be completely harmless if swallowed. Nowadays lipsticks do not usually stain.	Attractiveness depends a lot on the lips and eyes and hence special emphasis has always been given to suitable preparations which will appear to alter their colour or shape. At the same time the observer's attention is centred on these features.
5 Eye Preparations	Coloured solids, creams or liquids all of which have to be completely harmless to the eyes.	
6 Nail Varnish	Usually a shiny varnish but sometimes nylon or other chemical is added to strengthen the nails.	The hands are used a lot to express feelings and mood during conversation. Well-groomed nails add to the visual impact.

Manufacturing cosmetics

Many different departments with different skills and tasks are necessary for the production of successful and popular cosmetics. These are as follows:

Creativity section

Some products like Pond's Cold Cream seem to go on selling well, year in and year out, although many of its competitors are essentially similar. But many cosmetics are seasonal and what will sell splendidly this year will fail on the market next year. Partly this is due to changes in clothes fashions and colours. The **market research** members of the creativity department must keep themselves informed of the **fashions** to come and predict which colours will be fashionable in six months or a year's time.

Having predicted next season's main colours the **creator** dreams up a blending or contrasting colour scheme for the lips, eyes and nails. Obviously she hopes to launch a set of cosmetics which has novelty as well as being appropriate to the fashion. However, as she usually isn't a chemist she has to explain her ideas in another department, the laboratory section.

Laboratory section

It takes a lot of skill and experience to turn an idea into the reality of a new colour or texture. The chemist has some standard products to guide him so that when the creator says: 'I want a lipstick with a slightly purplish tinge of this pink', the chemist has a good starting point. By trial and error he then makes up several sets of colours and passes these back to the creator for comment. Eventually he will hit on the right colour and this will then be submitted to a meeting of the top executives of the firm for discussion and approval.

It's very rare indeed that anyone has a completely new idea — comb-on mascara was one. Nevertheless, the research and development section are working all the time on new mixtures of raw materials in the hope that something will come to light. Apart from this side of their work they are responsible for:

1. Working out the **formula** for each product and sending this to the factory.
2. **Checking** that samples from the factory are manufactured according to the given formula.
3. Making sure that suitable **preservatives** are used to keep all products in good condition on the shop shelf.
4. Making sure that all products are safe to use. Normally this means checking that all chemicals delivered to the factory are pure and exactly what they should be. If a chemical is being used for the first time ever, then testing would have to be done under hospital control but this is quite exceptional.
5. Checking advertising material to see that no false claims are made about products. For example, if a lotion is said to protect the skin against sunburn then it must do so.
6. Where products are going overseas, particularly to hot climates, then additional precautions have to be taken with regard to temperature, high humidity, packaging for travel and so on.

Obviously the research and development departments are tremendously important to the success of the firm's products.

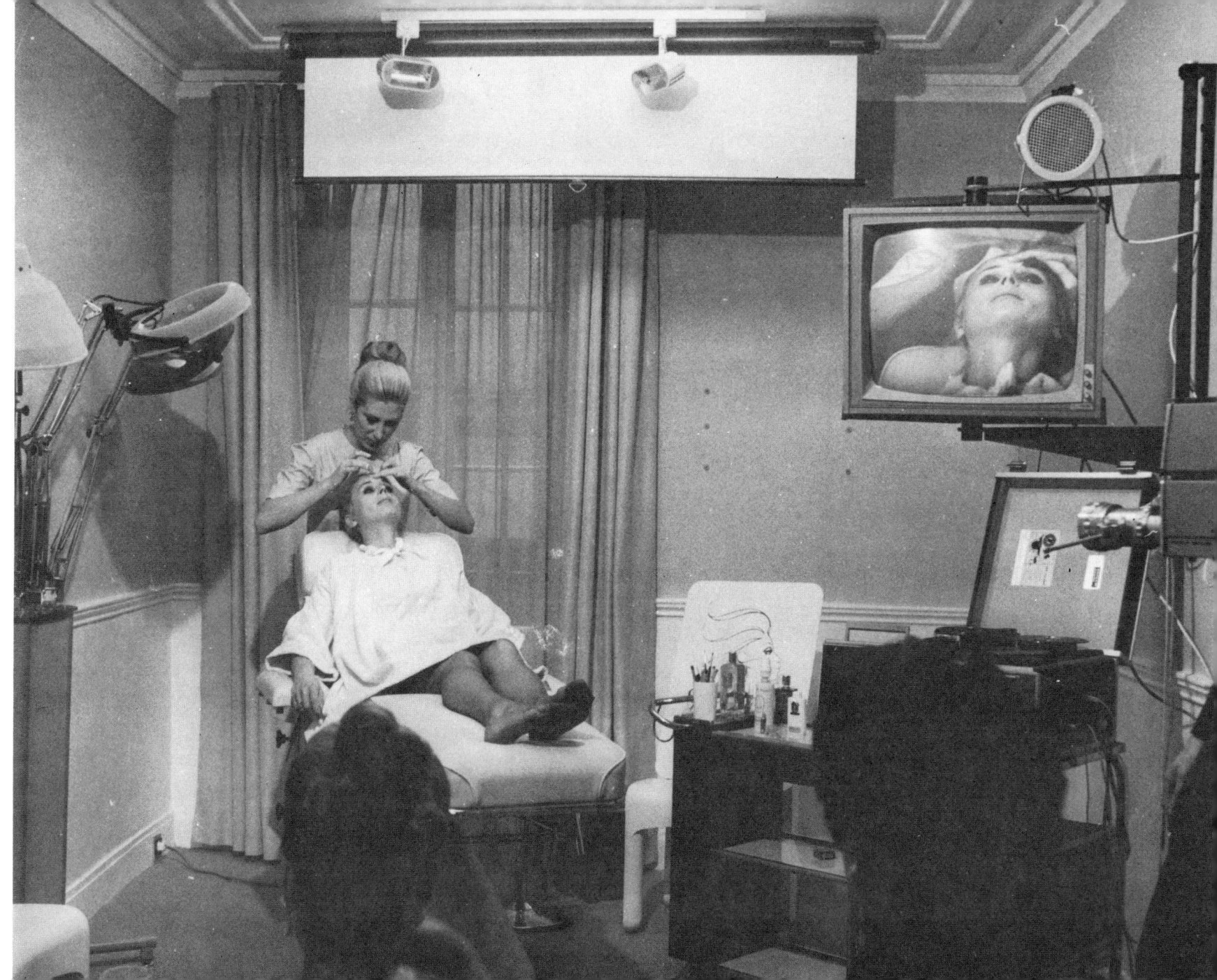

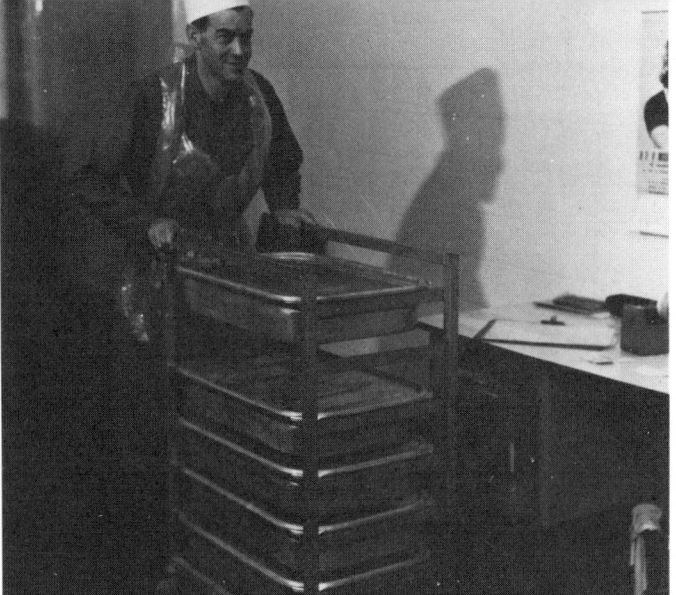
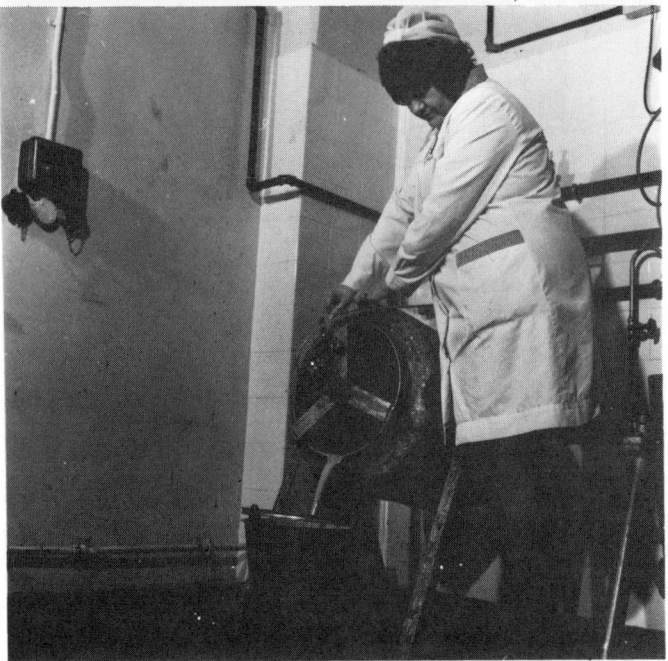

Factory

One often thinks that modern factories are working on an automatic basis and it is surprising to find so many workers on the production line in a cosmetics factory. The fact is that because many cosmetic lines are seasonal the quantities are relatively small and an automatic process would be uneconomic. Also, the containers of things like nail varnish come in all shapes and sizes so that one machine would have to be very complex if it were to deal with each container efficiently. The human hand is more versatile.

Manufacture of lipstick

Let's follow the production of a lipstick. What is most noticeable is the **cleanliness** and purity of everything to do with the production.

In the cauldrons
The first room is rather like the kitchen of a large canteen and one finds a row of huge cauldrons, each stirred automatically and each heated by a surrounding thermostatically controlled jacket. Carefully measured quantities of each component of the lipstick are taken from the stores and put into the cauldron; the stirrer is switched on and continues to stir until all the ingredients are completely blended together. Sometimes this batch may not be used for several weeks and so it is poured into a mould and blocks are made which can be stored or taken to another factory.

Filling the moulds
Some time later the blocks are melted in another cauldron and the liquid lipstick is poured into a controlled temperature hopper. From this, moulds are filled which, after cooling can be split to release the bullet-shaped lipstick. Obviously, in a hand operation of this kind many are slightly mis-shaped and these are picked out and re-melted. The perfect ones are sent to a production line where they are manually put into plastic holders.

In order to remove the handling marks and to give a glossy finish the mounted lipstick is passed through gas flames on a conveyor belt; the time of passage through the flames and the size of the flames are carefully adjusted so that there is no serious melting of the stick.

Ready for the shop
Beyond the flame another operator takes the lipstick in its holder and adds a screw-on cap after which it is labelled and boxed-up ready for the shop. Some lipstick production has been automated to some extent but the particular line has to be in high demand in order to warrant it.

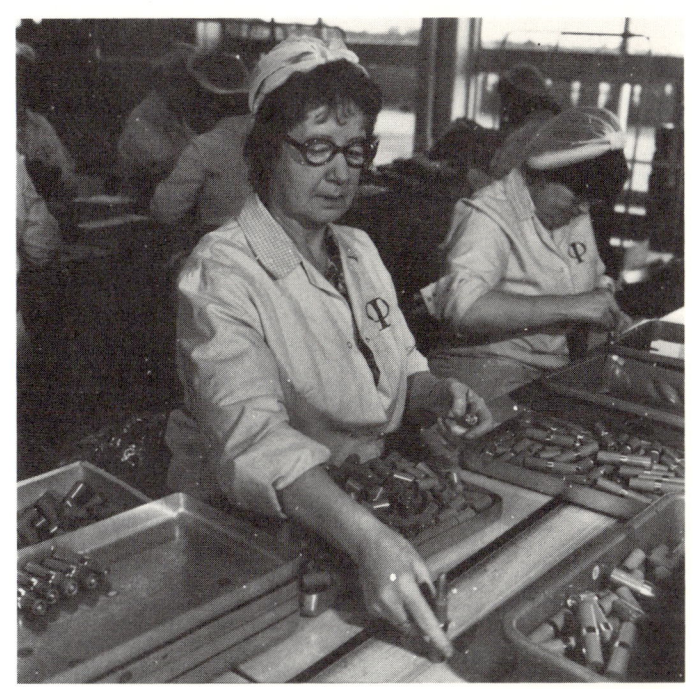

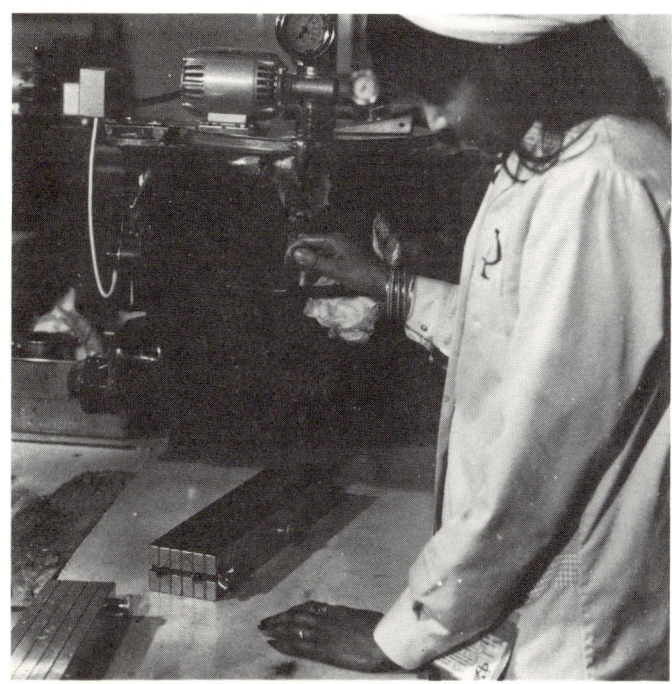

Processes in the factory: moving the blocks (*opposite, top*); pouring melted lipstick out from the hopper (*opposite, bottom*); filling the moulds (*left*); and checking finished lipsticks (*above*).

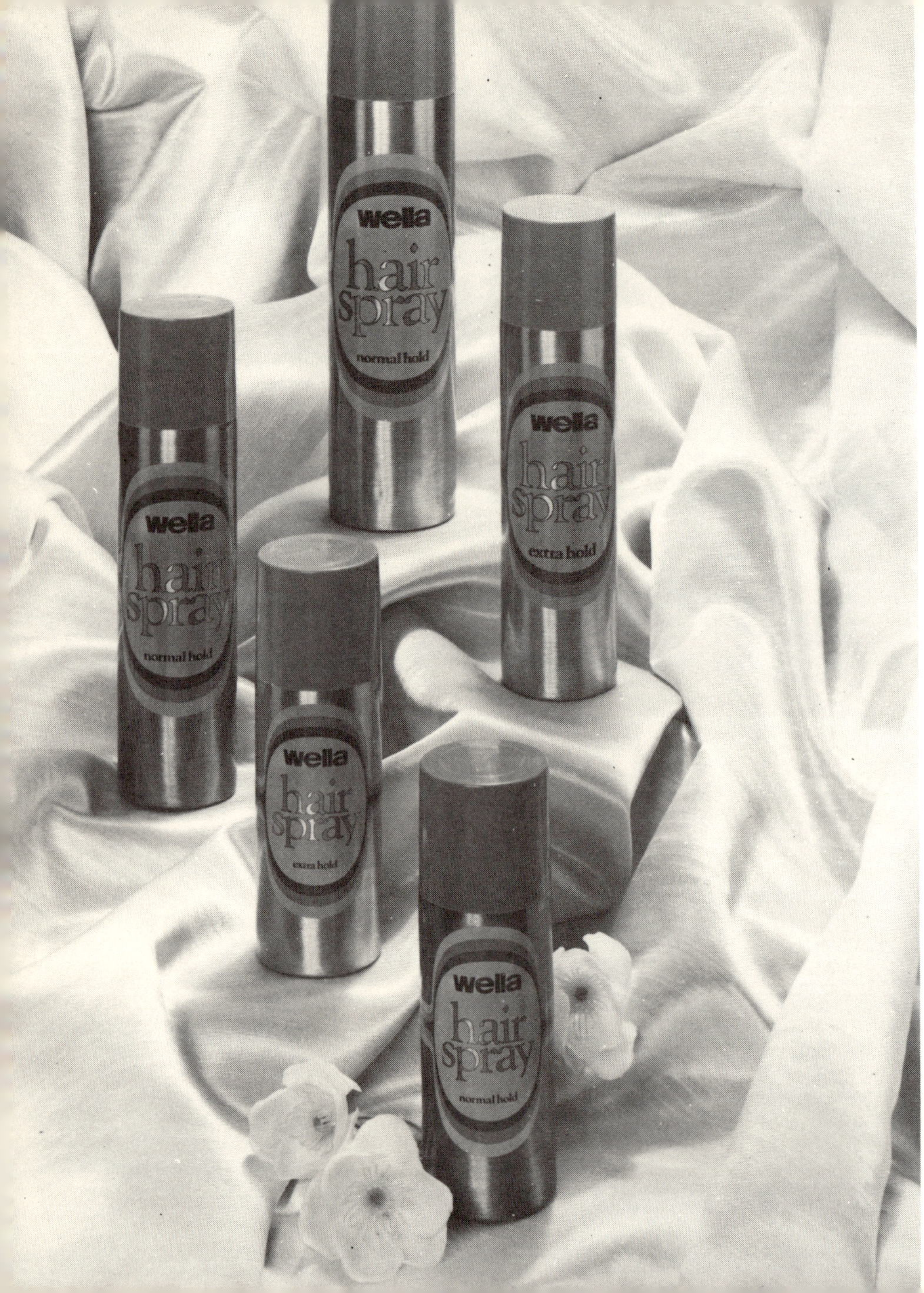

Package design department

What makes one type of cosmetic sell better than another? One reason could be that it is really of a superior quality with, maybe, a very exclusive scent. Another reason might be that the product is cheaper than its competitors. But all producers are vying with each other and are trying to get you to be their customer so that it is unusual for a manufacturer to charge more for his product than he is forced to do.

No, quality and price are important but **presentation of products** and **advertising** have a very definite influence on a person's choice. After twenty-five, women tend to settle down into the use of one or two particular lines and are then less influenced by the smart pack on the dressing table or eye-catching display in the shop. Because this side of the business is so important cosmetic firms employ lively minded people to design new shapes for bottles or lipstick holders, specially conspicuous and attractive boxes for shops, original colours and labelling.

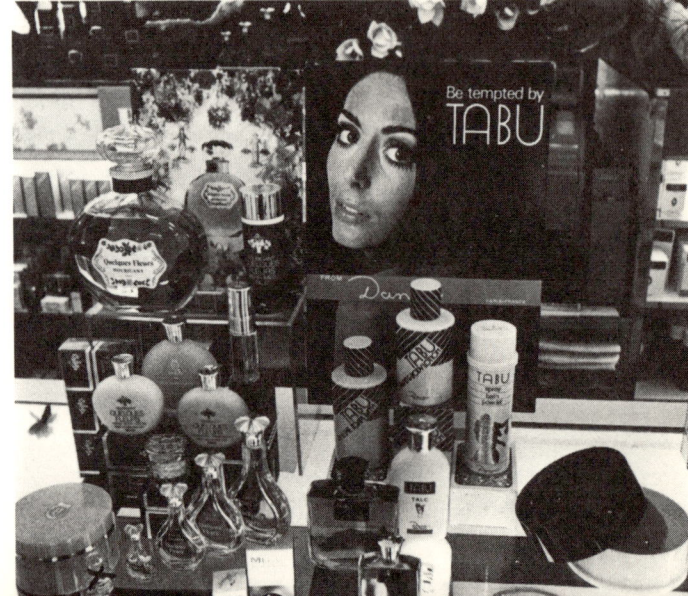

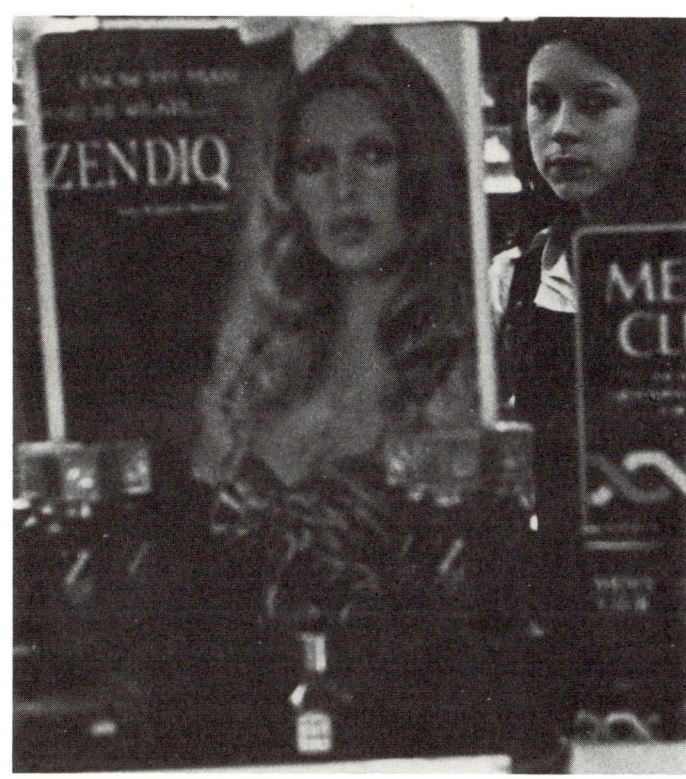

Next time you are in a chemist or large store go to the cosmetic department and look around at the displays. Most cosmetics are basically quite cheap to make but research and their packaging multiplies their costs many times over.

Psychologically we are all at our best if we feel that we are looking our best. Cosmetic production is a major industry these days to help people do just this and as more men become conscious of their general appearance so the industry will grow. Products range in price to cater for the early teenager to the wealthy and elderly but everything, cheap or exclusive, is designed to help you make the most of yourself.

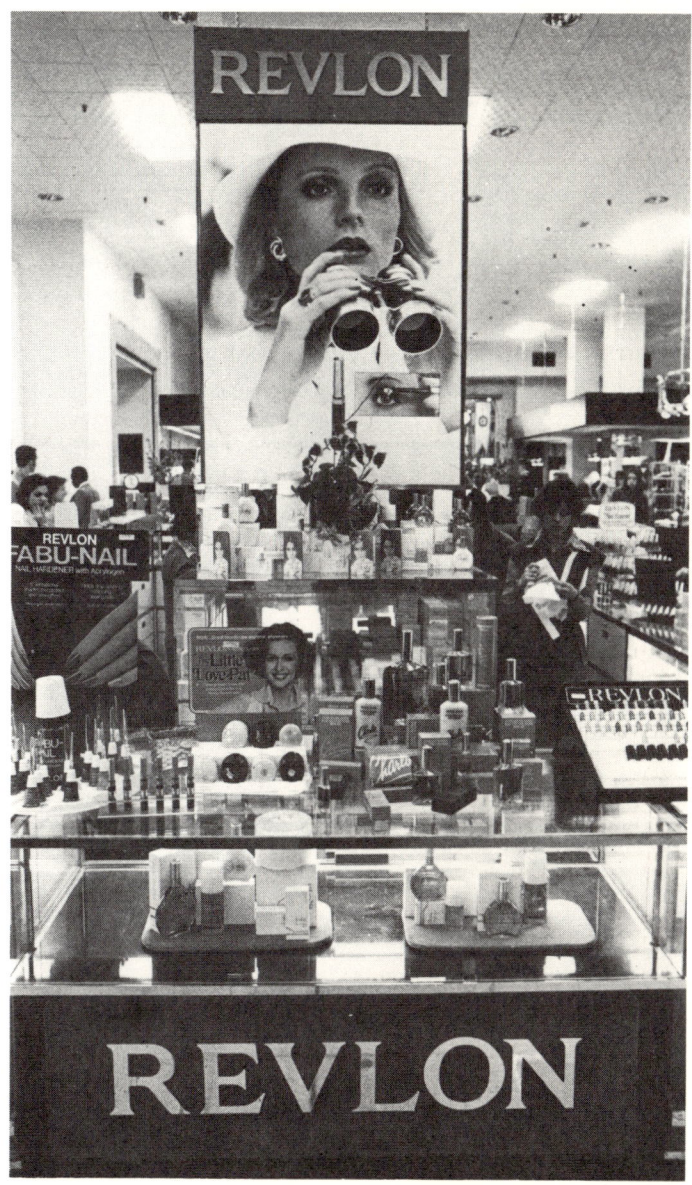

Things to do

1 Look up history books covering ancient Egypt and Elizabethan England. How did the men and women decorate themselves in those times? Was there a standard pattern or were people all different? Remember that the pictures you find will be of people from high society.

2 Visit a large store which sells cosmetics and make a list of all the different types of cosmetics which you can find on the shelves. Now count up all the shades of colour of lipstick and eye shadow. Are you surprised?

3 Next autumn or spring go to a large store selling fashionable clothes and find out which are the season's colours and styles. Now go to the cosmetics counters and see if there are corresponding colours and styles.

4 In 1945 very few men used cosmetics: go to the shops and make a list of what men are using now. Do you think men will use any other forms of cosmetics in the future which are not in use now?

© A. R. Kenney 1978
First Published 1978
Reprinted 1979

ISBN 0 17 438334 7

Thomas Nelson & Sons Ltd
Lincoln Way Windmill Road
Sunbury-on-Thames
Middlesex TW16 7HP
P.O. Box 73146 Nairobi Kenya
P.O. Box 943 95 Church Street Kingston Jamaica
308–312 Lockhart Road Golden Coronation Building
2nd Floor Blk A Hong Kong
29 Jalan Bangau Singapore 28

Thomas Nelson (Australia) Ltd
19–39 Jeffcott Street West Melbourne Victoria 3003

Thomas Nelson & Sons (Canada) Ltd
81 Curlew Drive Don Mills Ontario

Thomas Nelson (Nigeria) Ltd
8 Ilupeju Bypass PMB 21303 Ikeja Lagos

Phototypeset by Filmtype Services Limited, Scarborough
Printed and bound in Hong Kong

Acknowledgements
Special thanks are due to the following for their help to the author in the preparation of this book:

Crystal Products Co. Ltd (Gala Cosmetic Group)
E. R. Holloway Ltd (Evette Cosmetics)
Michael Murnane, BA, ARPS (Photographer)

The Publishers gratefully acknowledge permission to reproduce the following photographs:–

Henry Grant (2, L); Elizabeth Photo Library (2, R); George Roger, Magnum (3, L); Radio Times Hulton Picture Library (3, R); Ron Chapman (4, L below); Keystone Press Limited (4, L above and 19); Bruce Coleman (4, R, 5 and 6 bottom); Biofotos (6 Top); Elida Limited (7); Mary Evans Picture Library (10); Helena Rubenstein (11); Joe Clarke (14, 23 L); The Mansell Collection (15); Michael Murnane and the Gala Cosmetic Group (20 and 21); Terry Williams (22 and 23, R); André Bernard Hair International (13).